CONTENTS

INTRODUCTION

Welcome to the comprehensive guide on the full liquid diet—a dietary approach designed to provide essential nutrients while maintaining a liquid consistency. Whether you're facing a specific medical condition, recovering from surgery, or seeking a temporary dietary plan, this book will serve as your roadmap to understanding, implementing, and thriving on a full liquid diet.

A full liquid diet offers a valuable solution for individuals who are unable to consume solid foods due to various reasons such as gastrointestinal issues, dental problems, swallowing difficulties, or as part of a prescribed medical treatment. By providing essential nutrients in a liquid form, this specialized diet ensures adequate nourishment while accommodating the unique needs and challenges individuals may face.

Throughout the pages of this book, we will delve into the definition and purpose of a full liquid diet, explore its role in medical treatment and recovery, and uncover its benefits and potential risks. We will differentiate the full liquid diet from other dietary plans, highlighting its distinct characteristics and applications. Additionally, we will identify specific medical conditions where a full liquid diet is recommended, drawing insights from medical professionals who have extensive experience in utilizing this dietary approach.

One of the key aspects we will explore is the importance of maintaining a nutritionally complete liquid menu. We will provide guidelines and strategies for creating balanced and nourishing liquid meals, ensuring that essential macronutrients, vitamins, and minerals are included. You will discover a diverse range of recipes for milk, yogurt, cream-based soups, broths, fruit and vegetable juices, protein shakes, gelatin, pudding, smoothies, and more. These recipes will not only satisfy your nutritional requirements but also tantalize your taste buds, bringing enjoyment and variety to your full liquid diet journey.

It is crucial to approach the full liquid diet with caution and under the guidance of healthcare professionals, who can tailor the dietary plan to your specific needs and monitor your progress. This book aims to empower you with the knowledge and resources necessary to navigate the full liquid diet successfully. We will provide practical tips, meal planning strategies, and sample menus to accommodate different dietary needs and preferences, ensuring that you have the tools to achieve your health goals.

By immersing yourself in the wealth of information presented in this book, you will gain a comprehensive understanding of the full liquid diet and its impact on your well-being. You will embark on a journey towards optimal nutrition, recovery, and improved health. Remember, the full liquid diet is not just a temporary measure but an opportunity to embrace a nourishing lifestyle that supports your overall wellness.

So, let's dive in and unlock the secrets of the full liquid diet together. Get ready to embark on a transformative dietary experience that will invigorate your body, mind, and spirit. Your health and well-being await you within these pages.

CHAPTER ONE

Definition and purpose of a full liquid diet

A full liquid diet is a type of dietary plan that consists of consuming only foods and beverages in a liquid or semi-liquid form. Unlike a regular diet that includes solid foods, a full liquid diet focuses on fluids and foods that can be easily liquefied or strained to create a liquid consistency. This type of diet typically excludes any solid foods, as well as foods with a thick or lumpy texture.

The purpose of a full liquid diet is primarily to provide adequate nutrition while minimizing the stress on the digestive system. It is commonly prescribed for individuals who have difficulty chewing, swallowing, or digesting solid foods due to certain medical conditions, surgeries, or recovery periods. The diet allows for easy digestion and absorption of essential nutrients, vitamins, and minerals.

Medical Conditions Requiring a Full Liquid Diet:

- Post-Surgical Recovery: Following certain surgeries, such as oral or gastrointestinal procedures, a full liquid diet may be prescribed during the initial stages of recovery to allow the surgical site to heal without the strain of solid foods.

- Gastrointestinal Disorders: Individuals with gastrointestinal conditions, such as Crohn's disease, ulcerative colitis, or diverticulitis, may benefit from a full liquid diet during flare-ups or periods of intestinal inflammation. It helps to rest the digestive system and alleviate symptoms.
- Dental Procedures: Dental surgeries, including tooth extractions, jaw surgeries, or oral injuries, often necessitate a temporary shift to a full liquid diet to prevent chewing or irritating the surgical area.
- Swallowing Difficulties: People with dysphagia, a swallowing disorder, may find it challenging to safely consume solid foods. A full liquid diet can provide them with necessary nutrition while reducing the risk of choking or aspiration.
- Weight Loss Programs: In some weight loss programs, a full liquid diet may be used as a short-term meal replacement plan to facilitate rapid weight loss. However, it is crucial to consult a healthcare professional before embarking on such a diet for weight loss purposes.

The benefits of a full liquid diet include:

- Adequate Nutrition: While the diet may restrict certain food textures, it can still provide essential nutrients, vitamins, and minerals necessary for the body's functioning and recovery.
- Easy Digestion: Liquids are generally easier for the digestive system to break down, allowing the body

- to absorb nutrients more efficiently.
- Hydration: Many liquid-based foods and beverages contribute to hydration, helping maintain fluid balance in the body.
- Reduced Gastrointestinal Strain: By avoiding solid foods, a full liquid diet can minimize stress on the digestive system, allowing it to heal and recover from certain medical conditions or procedures.
- Temporary Relief: For individuals with specific medical conditions, a full liquid diet can provide temporary relief from symptoms, allowing the body to heal and recover more effectively.

It is important to note that a full liquid diet is typically used for short periods, as prolonged restriction of solid foods may lead to nutritional deficiencies. It is essential to consult with a healthcare professional or registered dietitian before starting a full liquid diet to ensure it is appropriate for your specific condition and to receive guidance on meeting nutritional needs while on the diet.

The role of a full liquid diet in medical treatment or recovery

A full liquid diet plays a crucial role in medical treatment and recovery by providing essential nutrition while allowing the body to heal and recuperate. It is often recommended by healthcare professionals to manage specific medical conditions, aid in post-surgical recovery, or facilitate the healing process after certain procedures. Here are some key aspects of the role of a full liquid diet in medical treatment or recovery:

- Easy Digestion and Nutrient Absorption: One of the primary benefits of a full liquid diet is its ease of digestion. Liquid-based foods and beverages require less effort from the digestive system to break down compared to solid foods. This allows the body to absorb essential nutrients, including proteins, carbohydrates, fats, vitamins, and minerals, more efficiently. In medical conditions where the digestive system may be compromised, such as gastrointestinal disorders or post-surgical recovery, a full liquid diet helps ensure that patients receive adequate nutrition without placing additional strain on their digestive systems.
- Resting the Digestive System: In certain medical conditions, such as acute gastrointestinal illnesses or surgeries involving the gastrointestinal tract, a full liquid diet is often prescribed to give the digestive system a period of rest. By temporarily eliminating solid foods, the diet reduces the workload on the digestive system, allowing it to heal and recover. This rest can be particularly beneficial in cases of intestinal inflammation, digestive disorders, or after procedures that may cause temporary sensitivity

or trauma to the digestive tract.

- Preventing Dehydration: Many liquid-based foods and beverages in a full liquid diet provide hydration. Adequate hydration is essential for overall health and plays a vital role in the recovery process. By including fluids with high water content, such as clear soups, broths, juices, and smoothies, a full liquid diet helps maintain proper fluid balance in the body, preventing dehydration, which can be especially important during illness or recovery periods.

- Soft Texture and Swallowing Difficulties: In medical conditions where individuals have difficulty chewing or swallowing solid foods, a full liquid diet offers an alternative solution. It provides nourishment in a soft, easily swallowable form, reducing the risk of choking or aspiration. This can be beneficial for individuals with dysphagia (swallowing difficulties), temporomandibular joint (TMJ) disorders, or following oral surgeries, as it allows them to maintain adequate nutrition while minimizing the physical strain associated with consuming solid foods.

- Calming Inflammation and Promoting Healing: Certain medical conditions or procedures can cause inflammation or irritation in the body. A full liquid diet can help soothe and calm inflammation by providing easily digestible and gentle foods. By avoiding potentially irritating or difficult-to-digest solid foods, the diet supports the healing process by minimizing further inflammation and allowing the body to focus on repairing damaged tissues or organs.

It is important to note that a full liquid diet is typically used for a specific duration as directed by healthcare professionals. Prolonged adherence to a full liquid diet without appropriate medical supervision can lead to nutritional deficiencies. Therefore, it is crucial to consult with healthcare professionals, such as doctors or registered dietitians, who can assess individual needs, monitor progress, and provide guidance on transitioning back to a regular diet when appropriate.

Overall, the role of a full liquid diet in medical treatment or recovery is to provide adequate nutrition, support healing, and minimize strain on the digestive system. It serves as a valuable tool in managing specific medical conditions, facilitating post-surgical recovery, and promoting overall well-being during periods when solid foods may not be suitable or well-tolerated.

Understanding the Full Liquid Diet:

Explaining the concept of a full liquid diet

The concept of a full liquid diet revolves around consuming

foods and beverages that are in a liquid or semi-liquid form, while excluding solid foods. It is a specific dietary plan designed to provide essential nutrition while minimizing the strain on the digestive system. Let's delve into the key aspects of the concept of a full liquid diet:

- Definition and Exclusions: A full liquid diet involves consuming foods and beverages that are easily liquefied or strained to create a liquid consistency. It excludes foods with a solid or chunky texture, as well as those that require chewing. Examples of foods not included in a full liquid diet are whole fruits and vegetables, meats, grains, nuts, seeds, and dairy products in solid form.
- Liquid and Semi-Liquid Foods: A full liquid diet includes a variety of liquid and semi-liquid foods that can provide nutrition in an easily digestible form. These include clear liquids like water, broth, and herbal tea, as well as thicker fluids such as milk, milkshakes, fruit juices, vegetable juices, and cream-based soups. Other options may include strained or pureed fruits, vegetables, and yogurts.
- Nutritional Adequacy: While the texture of the foods may be altered, it is crucial to ensure that a full liquid diet provides adequate nutrition. The diet should include a balance of macronutrients (carbohydrates, proteins, and fats) and essential micronutrients (vitamins and minerals) to support overall health and well-being. This can

be achieved through the incorporation of various liquid foods that are rich in nutrients or through the addition of liquid supplements if needed.

- Temporary Nature: A full liquid diet is typically used for a specific period, often as part of a medical treatment plan or recovery process. It is not intended to be a long-term dietary solution. The duration of the diet varies depending on the individual's medical condition, the stage of recovery, or the recommendation of a healthcare professional. It is essential to follow the prescribed duration and transition back to a regular diet under medical guidance.
- Customization and Adaptation: The concept of a full liquid diet allows for some customization based on individual needs and preferences. While certain foods may be restricted due to their solid form, there is still room for creativity in creating liquid-based meals that are palatable and enjoyable. For example, soups and smoothies can be customized with a variety of ingredients, flavors, and spices to enhance taste and nutrition.
- Medical Supervision: It is crucial to undertake a full liquid diet under the guidance and supervision of healthcare professionals, such as doctors or registered dietitians. They can assess the specific medical needs, monitor progress, ensure nutritional adequacy, and provide recommendations or modifications as necessary. They may also help with meal planning, recipe ideas, and transitioning back to a regular diet when appropriate.
- Precautions and Considerations: While a full

liquid diet can be beneficial in certain medical situations, it may not be suitable for everyone. Individuals with specific medical conditions, nutritional deficiencies, or complex dietary needs should consult healthcare professionals before starting a full liquid diet. It is important to address any underlying health concerns, consider potential interactions with medications, and tailor the diet to meet individual requirements.

The concept of a full liquid diet aims to provide necessary nutrition while accommodating specific medical needs or conditions. It allows for the consumption of a wide range of liquids and semi-liquids, while temporary excluding solid foods. Proper implementation, nutritional balance, and medical supervision are key to ensuring the diet's effectiveness and maintaining overall health during the prescribed period.

Differentiating it from other dietary plans

Differentiating a full liquid diet from other dietary plans involves considering the specific characteristics and restrictions of each plan. Here are some key points of differentiation between a full liquid diet and other common dietary plans:

- Full Liquid Diet vs. Clear Liquid Diet: A clear liquid

diet is a more restrictive form of a liquid diet that only includes transparent or translucent liquids. It typically allows clear broth, water, fruit juices without pulp, clear sodas, and gelatin. In contrast, a full liquid diet expands the variety of allowed liquids to include thicker fluids such as milk, milkshakes, and cream-based soups. Full liquid diets provide more nutrients and a wider range of food options compared to clear liquid diets.

- Full Liquid Diet vs. Soft Diet: A soft diet includes foods that are easily chewed and digested, but it still includes solid foods. It is often recommended for individuals with dental problems, difficulty chewing, or swallowing issues. Unlike a full liquid diet, a soft diet allows for foods like cooked vegetables, soft fruits, tender meats, and cooked grains. While a full liquid diet focuses solely on liquids and liquid-like foods, a soft diet includes some solid foods that are easier to consume.

- Full Liquid Diet vs. Pureed Diet: A pureed diet involves blending or pureeing solid foods to a smooth consistency. It is commonly used for individuals with swallowing difficulties or those who require easier-to-swallow meals. While a pureed diet includes foods that are mashed or pureed, it still retains some texture. A full liquid diet, on the other hand, consists of completely liquid or strained foods without any solid components. Pureed foods may be part of a full liquid diet during the transition phase but are not the sole components of the diet.

- Full Liquid Diet vs. Regular Diet: A regular diet comprises a balanced intake of solid foods from various food groups. It includes solid proteins, grains, fruits, vegetables, and dairy products. Unlike a full liquid diet, a regular diet offers a wider range of textures, flavors, and nutritional options. It is the standard dietary approach for individuals without specific medical conditions or dietary restrictions.

- Full Liquid Diet vs. Fasting or Cleansing Diets: Fasting or cleansing diets involve temporary periods of limited or no food intake for detoxification or weight loss purposes. These diets typically restrict both solid and liquid foods, focusing on herbal teas, water, or specific cleansing beverages. While a full liquid diet restricts solid foods, its primary aim is to provide adequate nutrition during medical treatment or recovery, rather than fasting or cleansing purposes.

It is important to note that these different dietary plans serve distinct purposes and have varying levels of restrictions. Each plan should be chosen based on individual needs and under the guidance of healthcare professionals or registered dietitians who can provide personalized recommendations and ensure proper nutrition.

Benefits and potential risks

associated with the diet

Benefits of a Full Liquid Diet:

- Adequate Nutrition: Despite the exclusion of solid foods, a full liquid diet can still provide essential nutrients, vitamins, and minerals necessary for the body's functioning and recovery. By including a variety of liquids and liquid-like foods, individuals can receive adequate protein, carbohydrates, fats, vitamins, and minerals to support their nutritional needs.
- Easy Digestion and Absorption: Liquids are generally easier for the digestive system to break down compared to solid foods. By consuming a full liquid diet, the digestive system requires less effort to process the food, allowing for easier digestion and absorption of nutrients. This can be especially beneficial for individuals with digestive disorders or those recovering from surgeries where the digestive system needs time to heal.
- Hydration: Many liquid-based foods and beverages in a full liquid diet contribute to hydration. Proper hydration is essential for overall health and plays a vital role in various bodily functions. By incorporating fluids like water, clear broths, juices, and smoothies, individuals on a full liquid diet can help maintain fluid balance in the body.
- Reduced Gastrointestinal Strain: The absence of solid foods in a full liquid diet can minimize stress on the digestive system. This reduction in gastrointestinal strain can be beneficial

for individuals with gastrointestinal disorders, inflammation, or other conditions that may exacerbate symptoms when consuming solid foods.

- Temporary Relief: For individuals with specific medical conditions, a full liquid diet can provide temporary relief from symptoms. By eliminating solid foods that may aggravate their condition, the diet allows the body to heal and recover more effectively. Conditions such as diverticulitis, Crohn's disease, or dysphagia may benefit from a full liquid diet to alleviate symptoms and promote healing.

Potential Risks and Considerations of a Full Liquid Diet:

- Nutritional Deficiencies: While a full liquid diet can provide adequate nutrition when properly planned, there is a risk of certain nutrient deficiencies. Solid foods often contribute essential dietary fiber, which may be lacking in a full liquid diet. It is important to work closely with a healthcare professional or registered dietitian to ensure appropriate nutrient intake and consider the potential need for supplements.
- Limited Variety and Taste: Following a full liquid diet can result in a limited variety of foods and flavors. This can potentially lead to monotony and reduced enjoyment of meals. It is important to explore different options, incorporate various flavors, and seek creative recipes to ensure satisfaction and compliance with the diet.
- Psychological Impact: The absence of solid foods and the reliance on liquids alone may have

psychological effects, particularly for individuals who have a strong attachment to or enjoyment of eating solid foods. It is essential to address any emotional or psychological concerns and seek support if needed to maintain a positive mindset during the dietary restrictions.

- Transition Back to Solid Foods: The transition from a full liquid diet back to a regular diet requires careful planning and guidance from healthcare professionals. Sudden reintroduction of solid foods may cause digestive discomfort or difficulty. Gradual reintroduction is typically recommended to allow the digestive system to adapt and prevent potential complications.

- Not Suitable for Prolonged Use: A full liquid diet is intended for short-term use and should not be prolonged without medical supervision. Restricting solid foods for an extended period can result in nutritional imbalances and deficiencies. It is essential to follow the prescribed duration of the diet and work with healthcare professionals to determine when to transition to a more regular and varied diet.

It is crucial to consult with healthcare professionals or registered dietitians before initiating a full liquid diet. They can assess individual needs, monitor progress, provide personalized guidance, and address any potential risks or complications associated with the diet.

Medical Conditions Requiring a Full Liquid Diet: Identifying conditions where a full liquid diet is recommended

A full liquid diet may be recommended in various medical conditions or situations where the consumption of solid foods is limited or not well-tolerated. It is important to note that the decision to prescribe a full liquid diet should be made by healthcare professionals based on individual circumstances. Here are some common conditions where a full liquid diet may be recommended:

- Post-Surgery Recovery: After certain surgeries, particularly those involving the gastrointestinal tract or oral cavity, a full liquid diet may be prescribed during the initial phase of recovery. It allows the surgical site or gastrointestinal system to heal without the added strain of digesting solid foods. Common surgeries that may require a full liquid diet include gastrointestinal surgeries, jaw surgeries, and dental procedures.
- Gastrointestinal Disorders: Individuals with gastrointestinal disorders, such as Crohn's disease, ulcerative colitis, diverticulitis, or irritable bowel syndrome (IBS), may experience periods of flare-ups or increased symptoms. During these times, a full liquid diet can help reduce irritation and inflammation in the

digestive tract. It allows the gastrointestinal system to rest and heal while still providing necessary nutrition.

- Dysphagia: Dysphagia is a condition characterized by difficulty in swallowing. It can be caused by neurological disorders, stroke, throat or esophageal conditions, or muscle weakness. In cases of severe dysphagia, where solid foods pose a risk of choking or aspiration, a full liquid diet may be recommended. It ensures that individuals receive adequate nutrition in a form that is safe and easily swallowed.
- Dental or Oral Surgery: Following dental procedures or oral surgeries, such as tooth extraction, jaw wiring, or oral trauma, a full liquid diet may be advised. The diet allows the mouth and oral tissues to heal without the need for chewing or biting on solid foods. It provides nourishment while minimizing discomfort and protecting the surgical site.
- Acute Illness or Infection: During periods of acute illness or infection, individuals may experience loss of appetite, nausea, vomiting, or difficulty swallowing. In such cases, a full liquid diet can provide easily digestible and soothing nutrition. It helps maintain hydration and supports the body's immune system during the recovery process.
- Cancer Treatment: Some individuals undergoing cancer treatments, such as chemotherapy or radiation therapy, may experience side effects that affect their ability to eat solid foods. These side effects may include mouth sores, nausea, or difficulty swallowing. A full liquid diet can be

recommended to ensure adequate nutrition and hydration during the treatment period.

- Pre- and Post-Procedure Preparation: Before certain medical procedures, such as colonoscopy or gastrointestinal imaging, a full liquid diet may be prescribed to clear the digestive tract. This helps ensure optimal visualization during the procedure. Similarly, a full liquid diet may be recommended during the immediate post-procedure period to allow the digestive system to recover gradually.

It is important to note that the duration and specifics of a full liquid diet may vary depending on the individual's condition, medical history, and healthcare professional's recommendations. It is crucial to consult with a healthcare professional or registered dietitian to determine the appropriateness of a full liquid diet and to receive personalized guidance on its implementation and duration.

Insights from medical professionals on the diet's role in specific conditions

Insights from medical professionals provide valuable perspectives on the role of a full liquid diet in specific medical conditions. While individual recommendations may vary, here are some general insights:

- Post-Surgery Recovery: Medical professionals emphasize that a full liquid diet plays a crucial role in the early stages of post-surgery recovery. According to surgical teams, this diet helps prevent complications, such as wound dehiscence or anastomotic leaks, by reducing strain on the digestive system. It allows for healing of the surgical site while ensuring adequate hydration and nutrition. As the recovery progresses, medical professionals may recommend gradually transitioning to a soft diet before returning to a regular diet.

- Gastrointestinal Disorders: Gastroenterologists and dietitians recognize the value of a full liquid diet in managing acute flare-ups of gastrointestinal disorders. They explain that this diet minimizes bowel movement frequency, reduces abdominal discomfort, and provides the necessary nutrients without exacerbating symptoms. Medical professionals stress the importance of tailored nutrition plans for individuals with specific conditions to address their unique needs, dietary restrictions, and nutritional deficiencies.

- Dysphagia Management: Speech-language pathologists and dysphagia specialists highlight the role of a full liquid diet in dysphagia management. They explain that individuals with difficulty swallowing may be at risk of aspiration or choking when consuming solid foods. A full liquid diet ensures safer and more manageable intake, preventing complications and maintaining adequate hydration and nutrition. Medical professionals stress the need for close monitoring and ongoing assessment to determine the appropriate texture and consistency of the liquids based on each individual's swallowing capabilities.

- Cancer Treatment Support: Oncologists and oncology dietitians acknowledge the benefits of a full liquid diet in supporting individuals undergoing cancer treatments. They point out that cancer treatments, such as chemotherapy and radiation therapy, often cause gastrointestinal side effects like nausea, mouth sores, and taste changes, making it challenging to consume solid foods. A full liquid diet offers a way to maintain nutrition and hydration while minimizing discomfort during treatment. Medical professionals may recommend consuming nutrient-dense liquids, such as high-protein shakes or smoothies, to help meet increased nutritional needs during this time.

- Dental or Oral Surgery: Dentists and oral surgeons highlight the importance of a full liquid diet in the immediate aftermath of dental or oral surgery. They emphasize the need to avoid chewing or biting on solid foods to prevent damage to the surgical site and promote healing. A full liquid diet provides essential nutrients in a form that is easy to consume and reduces the risk of infection. Medical professionals typically recommend gradually transitioning from a full liquid diet to a soft diet as the oral tissues heal.

Medical professionals stress that the decision to prescribe a full liquid diet is made on a case-by-case basis, considering individual medical history, nutritional needs, and treatment goals. They emphasize the importance of close monitoring, regular communication, and collaborative care between patients, healthcare professionals, and registered dietitians to ensure optimal outcomes and adjust the diet plan as needed. Individualized guidance from medical professionals is essential for tailoring the diet to the specific needs of each patient and providing ongoing support throughout their treatment or recovery journey.

Crafting a Balanced Liquid Menu: Detailed guidelines for creating a nutritionally complete liquid menu

Creating a nutritionally complete liquid menu requires careful consideration of various factors to ensure that all essential nutrients are included. Here are some guidelines to help create a well-balanced and nutritionally complete liquid menu:

- Consult with a Healthcare Professional or Registered Dietitian: Before designing a liquid menu, it is crucial to consult with a healthcare professional or registered dietitian who can assess individual nutritional needs, medical conditions, and dietary restrictions. They can provide personalized recommendations and ensure that the menu meets specific requirements.
- Include a Variety of Liquid Sources: Incorporate a wide range of liquids to provide different nutrients and prevent monotony. This may include milk, yogurt, fortified plant-based milk alternatives, vegetable juices, fruit juices, broths, soups, smoothies, protein shakes, and nutritional supplements. Different liquids offer varying profiles of macronutrients, vitamins, and minerals, ensuring a more comprehensive nutrient intake.
- Ensure Sufficient Protein: Protein is essential for tissue repair, immune function, and overall health. Include protein-rich liquids such as milk, yogurt, fortified plant-based milk alternatives, protein shakes, or liquid nutritional supplements. Aim for a balanced distribution of protein throughout the day to support muscle maintenance and healing.
- Include Healthy Fats: Incorporate sources of healthy fats to provide energy and essential fatty acids. This can include adding oils (such as olive oil or flaxseed oil) to soups or smoothies, using full-fat dairy products or nut butters in recipes,

or including avocados in blended concoctions. Consider using fortified liquid supplements that provide essential fatty acids.

- Incorporate Complex Carbohydrates: While a full liquid diet restricts whole grains and fibrous carbohydrates, it is still important to include complex carbohydrates for sustained energy. Use sources such as fruit juices, vegetable juices, milk, yogurt, and smoothies that contain naturally occurring sugars and provide essential vitamins and minerals.
- Include a Spectrum of Vitamins and Minerals: Aim for a diverse intake of fruits and vegetables through juicing or blending to obtain a wide range of vitamins and minerals. Consider adding fortified nutritional supplements or liquid multivitamins to ensure adequate intake of essential nutrients. Consult with a healthcare professional or registered dietitian to determine individual supplementation needs.
- Monitor and Adjust Caloric Intake: Depending on the individual's nutritional needs and goals, the liquid menu should be designed to meet appropriate caloric requirements. This may involve calculating energy needs based on factors such as age, sex, weight, activity level, and medical condition. Adjust the portion sizes and number of liquid meals or snacks accordingly to achieve the desired caloric intake.
- Consider Texture Modifications: In some cases, individuals on a full liquid diet may require modified textures to ensure safety and ease of consumption. For example, using thickeners or

pureeing foods to a smooth consistency can be necessary for individuals with swallowing difficulties or dysphagia. Collaborate with a speech-language pathologist or dysphagia specialist to determine the appropriate texture modifications.

- Gradual Transition Plan: If the full liquid diet is intended for a specific period of time, collaborate with healthcare professionals to develop a gradual transition plan to reintroduce solid foods. This allows the digestive system to adapt and prevents digestive discomfort. The transition plan should be personalized based on individual needs and medical conditions.

- Regular Monitoring and Adjustments: Regularly monitor the individual's nutritional status, weight, and overall well-being. Adjust the liquid menu as needed based on changes in health, nutrient requirements, or feedback from the individual. Continual communication with healthcare professionals or registered dietitians ensures that the liquid menu remains nutritionally balanced and supports the individual's specific needs.

Remember that these guidelines provide general principles for creating a nutritionally complete liquid menu. Individual needs and preferences may vary, so it is essential to work closely with a healthcare professional or registered dietitian to tailor the liquid menu to specific requirements. They can provide ongoing support, monitor nutritional adequacy, and make adjustments as needed.

Additional Considerations:

- Hydration: Adequate hydration is vital for overall health. Encourage the consumption of water, herbal teas, clear broths, and other hydrating liquids throughout the day, in addition to the nutrient-rich liquids. Monitor fluid intake and adjust as necessary to maintain proper hydration.
- Texture and Variety: While a full liquid diet primarily consists of liquids, incorporating some variety in texture can enhance the sensory experience of eating. For example, including smoothies with small fruit pieces, thin pureed soups with added vegetable chunks, or strained soups with small pieces of meat or vegetables can add interest and satisfaction to the diet.
- Individual Preferences and Tolerance: Consider the individual's food preferences, taste preferences, and tolerance when creating the liquid menu. Adapt the menu to accommodate personal likes and dislikes, cultural considerations, and specific dietary restrictions, such as lactose intolerance or allergies. This helps to enhance compliance and enjoyment of the diet.
- Regular Monitoring and Support: Regular monitoring of weight, nutritional markers, and overall well-being is crucial. Conduct follow-up visits with healthcare professionals or registered dietitians to assess the individual's progress, address concerns, and make any necessary adjustments to the liquid menu. Ongoing support

and guidance are vital for long-term success.

- Education and Resources: Provide education and resources to the individual and their caregivers on the importance of following the liquid diet, proper food handling and preparation techniques, and strategies to maintain a balanced and enjoyable eating experience. This empowers individuals to actively participate in their nutritional care and promotes adherence to the prescribed liquid menu.

Remember that a nutritionally complete liquid menu is just one component of overall health and well-being. It is important to consider other aspects of a healthy lifestyle, such as physical activity, stress management, and sleep quality, in conjunction with the liquid diet to support optimal health outcomes.

Creating a nutritionally complete liquid menu requires careful planning, individualization, and collaboration with healthcare professionals. By addressing specific nutritional needs and preferences, monitoring progress, and making necessary adjustments, a well-balanced and nutritionally complete liquid menu can support individuals in achieving their health and recovery goals.

Varieties of liquid foods and their nutritional profiles

There are various varieties of liquid foods that can be incorporated into a liquid diet, each offering unique nutritional profiles. Here are some examples:

- Milk and Dairy Products: Milk, including cow's milk, soy milk, almond milk, or other fortified plant-based milk alternatives, is a common base for liquid meals. Dairy products such as yogurt and kefir can also be included. These liquids provide a good source of protein, calcium, vitamin D, and other essential vitamins and minerals.
- Fruit and Vegetable Juices: Freshly squeezed or commercially available fruit and vegetable juices are rich in vitamins, minerals, and antioxidants. They provide hydration and a wide range of nutrients depending on the fruits and vegetables used. Orange juice is a good source of vitamin C, while carrot juice provides vitamin A and beta-carotene.
- Soups and Broths: Clear or strained soups and broths made from vegetables, meats, or bone broth can be included in a liquid diet. These liquids provide hydration, flavor, and essential nutrients. Vegetable-based soups offer vitamins, minerals, and fiber, while meat or bone broths can provide additional protein and minerals.

- Protein Shakes and Smoothies: Protein shakes and smoothies are versatile options that can be customized with various ingredients. They often contain a liquid base, protein powder, and a combination of fruits, vegetables, nuts, seeds, or nut butter. Protein shakes provide a concentrated source of protein, while smoothies offer a range of vitamins, minerals, fiber, and antioxidants.

- Nutritional Supplements: Liquid nutritional supplements are specially formulated to provide a balanced blend of macronutrients and micronutrients. They are available in a variety of flavors and can be used as a convenient way to supplement the diet with additional calories, protein, vitamins, and minerals. Nutritional supplements should be chosen based on individual needs and recommendations from healthcare professionals.

- Meal Replacement Drinks: Meal replacement drinks are designed to provide a complete and balanced nutritional profile, usually in a convenient ready-to-drink format. They can be used as a substitute for a traditional meal and typically contain a balance of protein, carbohydrates, healthy fats, vitamins, and minerals. Meal replacement drinks can be useful in situations where solid food is not an option.

- Hydration Beverages: In addition to the nutrient-rich liquids mentioned above, hydration beverages such as water, herbal teas, clear broths, and electrolyte drinks are important for maintaining proper hydration. These liquids do not provide significant macronutrients but are essential for overall health and hydration balance. It is important to note that the nutritional profiles of these liquid foods may vary based on brand, preparation methods, and added ingredients. It is advisable to read labels, choose options without added sugars or artificial additives, and consult with healthcare professionals or registered dietitians to select the most appropriate liquids based on individual nutritional needs and dietary restrictions.

Meal planning strategies and sample menus for different dietary needs

Meal planning strategies and sample menus can be tailored to different dietary needs, ensuring that individuals receive proper nutrition while accommodating their specific requirements. Here are some strategies and sample menus for various dietary needs:

General Healthy Eating:

- Ensure a balance of macronutrients: Include a source of lean protein (such as chicken, fish, tofu, or legumes), complex carbohydrates (like whole grains or starchy vegetables), and healthy fats (such as avocado, nuts, or olive oil) in each meal.

- Incorporate a variety of fruits and vegetables: Aim for a colorful mix of fruits and vegetables to provide a range of vitamins, minerals, and antioxidants.
- Portion control: Practice portion control by using appropriate serving sizes and balancing calorie intake with energy expenditure.

Sample Menu:

- Breakfast: Greek yogurt with mixed berries and a sprinkle of granola.
- Snack: Carrot sticks with hummus.
- Lunch: Grilled chicken breast with quinoa and roasted vegetables.
- Snack: Apple slices with almond butter.
- Dinner: Baked salmon with sweet potato and steamed broccoli.
- Dessert: Mixed fruit salad.

Vegetarian or Vegan:

- Ensure plant-based protein sources: Include legumes, tofu, tempeh, seitan, quinoa, or plant-based protein powders in meals to meet protein needs.
- Incorporate a variety of plant-based fats: Use sources such as avocado, nuts, seeds, and plant-based oils (like olive oil or coconut oil) to obtain healthy fats.
- Include fortified foods: Ensure sufficient intake of nutrients like vitamin B12, iron, and calcium by incorporating fortified plant-based milk alternatives, nutritional yeast, and leafy greens.

Sample Menu:

- Breakfast: Oatmeal topped with almond milk, berries, and walnuts.
- Snack: Edamame.
- Lunch: Chickpea salad wrap with mixed greens and tahini dressing.
- Snack: Veggie sticks with guacamole.
- Dinner: Stir-fried tofu with vegetables and brown rice.
- Dessert: Vegan dark chocolate mousse made with avocado and cocoa powder.

Gluten-Free:

- Focus on naturally gluten-free foods: Emphasize foods like fruits, vegetables, lean proteins, dairy products, nuts, seeds, and gluten-free grains (such as rice, quinoa, and oats labeled gluten-free).
- Read labels: Pay attention to food labels and avoid products that contain gluten or are processed in facilities that handle gluten-containing ingredients.

Sample Menu:

- Breakfast: Gluten-free oatmeal with almond milk, sliced banana, and chia seeds.
- Snack: Rice cakes with almond butter.
- Lunch: Grilled chicken or salmon salad with mixed greens, vegetables, and a gluten-free vinaigrette.
- Snack: Greek yogurt with gluten-free granola.
- Dinner: Grilled steak with roasted sweet potatoes and steamed vegetables.

- Dessert: Gluten-free chocolate chip cookies made with almond flour.

Diabetic-Friendly:

- Choose low glycemic index (GI) foods: Opt for whole grains, non-starchy vegetables, lean proteins, and healthy fats to help manage blood sugar levels.
- Monitor carbohydrate intake: Control portion sizes of carbohydrate-rich foods and spread them evenly throughout the day.
- Emphasize fiber-rich foods: Include plenty of fiber from vegetables, fruits, whole grains, legumes, and nuts to promote steady blood sugar levels.

Sample Menu:

- Breakfast: Veggie omelet with spinach, bell peppers, and feta cheese.
- Snack: Celery sticks with peanut butter.
- Lunch: Grilled chicken or fish with quinoa and steamed broccoli.
- Snack: Greek yogurt with mixed berries.
- Dinner: Baked salmon with roasted Brussels sprouts and a side salad with vinaigrette dressing.
- Dessert: Sugar-free Jello with whipped cream.

Heart-Healthy:

- Focus on lean proteins: Choose lean cuts of meat, skinless poultry, fish, legumes, and tofu as protein sources to reduce saturated fat intake.
- Include healthy fats: Incorporate sources of monounsaturated and polyunsaturated fats, such

as avocados, nuts, seeds, olive oil, and fatty fish, to support heart health.

- Reduce sodium intake: Limit processed foods, canned soups, and condiments high in sodium. Opt for fresh herbs, spices, and homemade dressings to add flavor.

Sample Menu:

- Breakfast: Veggie and egg white scramble with whole grain toast and sliced avocado.
- Snack: Almonds and an apple.
- Lunch: Grilled chicken or shrimp salad with mixed greens, cherry tomatoes, cucumber, and a lemon vinaigrette.
- Snack: Greek yogurt with a sprinkle of flaxseeds.
- Dinner: Baked salmon with quinoa and roasted asparagus.
- Dessert: Fresh mixed berries with a dollop of Greek yogurt.

Renal-Friendly:

- Limit sodium and potassium: Reduce salt intake and choose low-sodium alternatives. Limit high-potassium foods like bananas, oranges, and tomatoes.
- Control phosphorus intake: Avoid foods high in phosphorus, such as dairy products, processed meats, and colas. Choose lower phosphorus alternatives.
- Monitor protein intake: Adjust protein intake based on individual needs. Opt for high-quality protein sources like lean meats, eggs, and fish.

Sample Menu:

- Breakfast: Egg white omelet with spinach, mushrooms, and low-sodium cheese.
- Snack: Rice cakes with almond butter.
- Lunch: Grilled chicken breast with quinoa and steamed green beans.
- Snack: Low-potassium fruit salad (berries, grapes, and apples).
- Dinner: Baked white fish with lemon, steamed carrots, and a side salad with low-phosphorus dressing.
- Dessert: Sugar-free gelatin.

Remember to adapt these sample menus to individual preferences, portion sizes, and specific dietary requirements. It is always recommended to consult with a healthcare professional or registered dietitian to create a meal plan tailored to your specific needs. They can provide personalized guidance and ensure that nutritional goals are met while considering any underlying health conditions or medications.

CHAPTER TWO

Milk Recipe:

Ingredients:

- 2 cups of cow's milk, soy milk, almond milk, or any milk of your choice

Instructions:

- Pour the milk into a small saucepan.
- Place the saucepan over medium heat and slowly bring the milk to a gentle simmer. Stir occasionally to prevent scorching.
- Once the milk reaches a simmer, reduce the heat to low and continue simmering for about 5 minutes.
- Remove the saucepan from the heat and let the milk cool slightly before consuming or using it in other recipes.
- If desired, you can add a sweetener like honey or sugar, or flavorings such as vanilla extract or cocoa powder to enhance the taste.

Yogurt Recipe:

Ingredients:

- 4 cups of milk (cow's milk, soy milk, almond milk, etc.)

- 2 tablespoons of plain yogurt with live and active cultures (as a starter)

Instructions:

- Pour the milk into a large saucepan and heat it over medium heat until it reaches a temperature of around 180°F (82°C). Stir occasionally to prevent scorching.
- Remove the saucepan from heat and let it cool to about 110°F (43°C). Use a thermometer to measure the temperature.
- Once the milk has cooled, spoon the plain yogurt with live and active cultures into a small bowl.
- Take a ladleful of warm milk and mix it thoroughly with the yogurt in the bowl to temper the yogurt.
- Pour the tempered yogurt mixture back into the saucepan with the remaining milk. Stir gently to combine.
- Cover the saucepan with a clean towel or plastic wrap and place it in a warm spot, like an oven with the light on or a yogurt maker, for about 6-8 hours. This allows the mixture to ferment and thicken into yogurt.
- After the incubation period, refrigerate the yogurt for a few hours to chill and set completely before consuming. You can add sweeteners, fruits, or flavorings to the yogurt if desired.

Cream-based Soup Recipe:

Ingredients:

- 2 cups of vegetable or chicken broth
- 1 cup of chopped vegetables (such as carrots, celery, or broccoli)
- 1 tablespoon of butter or olive oil
- 1 tablespoon of all-purpose flour
- 1 cup of milk (cow's milk, soy milk, almond milk, etc.)
- Salt and pepper to taste

Instructions:

- In a saucepan, heat the butter or olive oil over medium heat.
- Add the chopped vegetables and sauté them for a few minutes until they become tender.
- Sprinkle the flour over the vegetables and stir well to coat them.
- Slowly pour in the vegetable or chicken broth while stirring continuously to avoid lumps.
- Bring the mixture to a simmer and let it cook for about 10-15 minutes, or until the vegetables are fully cooked and soft.
- Reduce the heat to low and gradually stir in the milk. Continue cooking for another 5 minutes, stirring occasionally.
- Season the soup with salt and pepper to taste.
- Remove the soup from heat and let it cool slightly.
- Use an immersion blender or regular blender to puree the soup until smooth and creamy.
- If desired, you can strain the soup through a fine-mesh sieve to achieve a smoother texture.
- Reheat the soup if necessary before serving. Adjust the seasoning if needed.

Broth Recipe:

Ingredients:

- 4 cups of water
- 1 pound of chicken bones, beef bones, or vegetables (depending on the desired broth)
- 1 onion, chopped
- 2 carrots, chopped
- 2 celery stalks, chopped
- Salt and pepper to taste

Instructions:

- In a large pot, combine the water, bones (if using), onion, carrots, celery, salt, and pepper.
- Bring the mixture to a boil over high heat.
- Once boiling, reduce the heat to low and let the broth simmer for about 1-2 hours to allow the flavors to develop.
- Skim off any foam or impurities that rise to the surface during simmering.
- After the simmering time, remove the pot from heat and strain the broth using a fine-mesh sieve or cheesecloth to separate the solids from the liquid.
- Discard the solids and let the broth cool before storing it in airtight containers in the refrigerator or freezer.
- The broth can be used as a base for soups, stews, or consumed on its own.

Fruit Juice Recipe:

Ingredients:

- 4-5 medium-sized apples, oranges, or grapes (or a combination of fruits)
- Water (optional, to adjust the consistency)
- Sweetener (optional, to taste)

Instructions:

- Wash and prepare the fruits by removing any stems, seeds, or peels.
- Cut the fruits into smaller pieces for easier juicing.
- Using a juicer or a blender, extract the juice from the fruits. If using a blender, blend the fruits until smooth and strain the mixture through a fine-mesh sieve or cheesecloth to separate the pulp.
- If desired, you can add water to the juice to adjust the consistency and dilute the flavor.
- Taste the juice and add sweetener (such as honey or sugar) if desired, depending on the sweetness of the fruits used.
- Stir well to ensure the sweetener is fully dissolved.
- Chill the fruit juice in the refrigerator before serving, or serve it over ice.

Vegetable Juice Recipe:

Ingredients:

- 3-4 medium-sized carrots

- 2 tomatoes
- 1 small beet
- Water (optional, to adjust the consistency)
- Lemon juice (optional, for added flavor)

Instructions:

- Wash and peel the carrots, tomatoes, and beet.
- Cut the vegetables into smaller pieces for easier juicing.
- Using a juicer or a blender, extract the juice from the vegetables. If using a blender, blend the vegetables until smooth and strain the mixture through a fine-mesh sieve or cheesecloth to remove any solids or pulp.
- If the juice is too concentrated or thick, you can add water to adjust the consistency.
- Optionally, add a squeeze of lemon juice for added flavor and freshness.
- Stir well to combine the ingredients.
- Chill the vegetable juice in the refrigerator before serving, or serve it over ice.

Protein Shake/Smoothie Recipe:

Ingredients:

- 1 cup of milk (cow's milk, soy milk, almond milk, etc.)
- 1/2 cup of plain yogurt or Greek yogurt
- 1 scoop of protein powder (flavor of your choice)
- 1 ripe banana
- 1 tablespoon of nut butter (peanut butter, almond

butter)
- Ice cubes (optional, for a chilled and thicker consistency)
- Sweetener (optional, to taste)

Instructions:

- In a blender, combine the milk, yogurt, protein powder, ripe banana, nut butter, and ice cubes (if using).
- Blend the ingredients until smooth and creamy.
- Taste the mixture and add sweetener (such as honey, maple syrup, or stevia) if desired, adjusting the sweetness to your liking.
- Blend again briefly to incorporate the sweetener.
- Pour the protein shake/smoothie into a glass and serve immediately.

Gelatin Recipe:

Ingredients:

- 1 package of gelatin powder (plain or fruit-flavored)
- 2 cups of water
- Sweetener (optional, to taste)

Instructions:

- In a small saucepan, combine the gelatin powder and water.
- Let the mixture sit for a few minutes to allow the gelatin to soften.
- Place the saucepan over low heat and stir

continuously until the gelatin is completely dissolved.

- If desired, add sweetener (such as sugar or artificial sweetener) to the mixture, adjusting the sweetness to your preference. Stir well to dissolve the sweetener.
- Remove the saucepan from heat and let the gelatin mixture cool slightly.
- Pour the mixture into individual serving cups or a large mold.
- Place the cups or mold in the refrigerator and let the gelatin set for a few hours or according to the package instructions.
- Once set, the gelatin is ready to be served. You can enjoy it as is or top it with fruits, whipped cream, or a sauce of your choice.

Pudding Recipe:

Ingredients:

- 2 cups of milk (cow's milk, soy milk, almond milk, etc.)
- 1/4 cup of sugar
- 1/4 cup of cornstarch
- 2 tablespoons of unsweetened cocoa powder (for chocolate pudding) or 1 teaspoon of vanilla extract (for vanilla pudding)
- Pinch of salt

Instructions:

- In a saucepan, combine the milk, sugar,

cornstarch, cocoa powder (for chocolate pudding) or vanilla extract (for vanilla pudding), and salt.

- Place the saucepan over medium heat and whisk the mixture continuously until it thickens and comes to a boil.
- Reduce the heat to low and let the pudding simmer for an additional 2 minutes, stirring constantly.
- Remove the saucepan from heat and let the pudding cool slightly.
- Pour the pudding into individual serving cups or a large bowl.
- Cover the pudding with plastic wrap, making sure the wrap touches the surface of the pudding to prevent a skin from forming.
- Chill the pudding in the refrigerator for at least 2 hours or until it is fully set.
- Serve the pudding chilled, either on its own or with toppings such as whipped cream, fruits, or sprinkles.

Fruit Smoothie Recipe:

Ingredients:

- 1 cup of frozen fruits (such as berries, mangoes, pineapples, or peaches)
- 1/2 cup of plain yogurt or Greek yogurt
- 1/2 cup of milk (cow's milk, soy milk, almond milk, etc.)
- 1 tablespoon of honey or maple syrup (optional, for added sweetness)
- Ice cubes (optional, for a chilled and thicker

consistency)

Instructions:

- In a blender, combine the frozen fruits, yogurt, milk, and sweetener (if using).
- Blend the ingredients on high speed until smooth and creamy.
- If the smoothie is too thick, you can add a few ice cubes and blend again to achieve the desired consistency.
- Taste the smoothie and adjust the sweetness by adding more sweetener if desired.
- Blend briefly to incorporate the added sweetener.
- Pour the fruit smoothie into a glass and serve immediately.

Ice Cream or Sorbet Recipe:

Ingredients:

- 2 cups of frozen fruits (such as bananas, strawberries, or mangoes)
- 1/2 cup of milk (cow's milk, soy milk, almond milk, etc.)
- 1-2 tablespoons of sweetener (such as honey, maple syrup, or sugar) - optional, depending on the sweetness of the fruits

Instructions:

- In a blender or food processor, combine the frozen fruits and milk.
- Blend the mixture on high speed, stopping

occasionally to scrape down the sides, until the ingredients are well combined and have a creamy consistency.

- If desired, add sweetener to the mixture and blend again to incorporate the sweetness.
- Taste the ice cream or sorbet base and adjust the sweetness as needed.
- Transfer the mixture to a freezer-safe container and freeze it for at least 2-3 hours, or until it reaches a firm consistency.
- Remove the container from the freezer and let the ice cream or sorbet soften slightly before scooping and serving.

Fruit Puree Recipe:

Ingredients:

- 2 cups of fruits (such as apples, bananas, or peaches)
- Water (optional, for thinning the puree)

Instructions:

- Wash, peel, and core the fruits as needed.
- Cut the fruits into small pieces.
- Place the fruit pieces in a blender or food processor.
- Blend the fruits until they reach a smooth and pureed consistency.
- If the puree is too thick, you can add a small amount of water to thin it to your desired consistency.

- Blend again briefly to incorporate the water if added.
- Taste the fruit puree and adjust the sweetness if desired, by adding a small amount of sweetener like honey or sugar.
- Blend briefly to incorporate the sweetener.
- Transfer the fruit puree to a container and refrigerate it until ready to serve.
- The fruit puree can be enjoyed on its own, used as a topping for desserts, or incorporated into other recipes

Mashed Potatoes:

Ingredients:

- 2 large potatoes, peeled and cubed
- 1/4 cup of milk (cow's milk, soy milk, almond milk, etc.)
- 2 tablespoons of unsalted butter or margarine
- Salt and pepper to taste

Instructions:

- Place the potatoes in a large pot and cover them with water.
- Bring the pot to a boil over medium heat and cook the potatoes until they are tender when pierced with a fork (approximately 15-20 minutes).
- Drain the cooked potatoes and return them to the pot.
- Add the milk and butter to the pot.
- Use a potato masher or an electric mixer to mash the potatoes until they reach a smooth and

creamy consistency.
- Season the mashed potatoes with salt and pepper to taste.
- Stir well to incorporate the seasoning.
- Serve the mashed potatoes hot.

Carrot Puree:

Ingredients:

- 4 large carrots, peeled and sliced
- 1/2 cup of vegetable broth or water
- 2 tablespoons of unsalted butter or olive oil
- Salt and pepper to taste

Instructions:

- Place the sliced carrots and vegetable broth (or water) in a saucepan.
- Bring the liquid to a boil over medium heat.
- Reduce the heat to low, cover the saucepan, and let the carrots simmer until they are very tender (approximately 15-20 minutes).
- Drain the cooked carrots, reserving the liquid.
- Transfer the carrots to a blender or food processor.
- Add the butter or olive oil to the blender along with a small amount of the reserved cooking liquid.
- Blend the carrots until they reach a smooth and creamy consistency, adding more of the reserved liquid if needed to achieve the desired thickness.
- Season the carrot puree with salt and pepper to taste.

- Blend again briefly to incorporate the seasoning.
- Serve the carrot puree hot or warm.

Nut Butter Recipe:

Ingredients:

- 2 cups of nuts (peanuts for peanut butter, almonds for almond butter)
- Salt (optional, to taste)
- Sweetener (optional, such as honey or sugar, to taste)

Instructions:

- Preheat the oven to 350°F (175°C).
- Spread the nuts evenly on a baking sheet.
- Roast the nuts in the oven for about 10-15 minutes until they are fragrant and lightly golden. Keep an eye on them to prevent burning.
- Remove the nuts from the oven and let them cool for a few minutes.
- Transfer the roasted nuts to a food processor or a high-speed blender.
- Blend the nuts, scraping down the sides occasionally, until they reach a smooth and creamy consistency. This may take several minutes, depending on the power of your blender or processor.
- If desired, add a pinch of salt and a small amount of sweetener (such as honey or sugar) to enhance the flavor. Blend again to incorporate the seasoning.

- Taste the nut butter and adjust the salt and sweetener according to your preference.
- Transfer the nut butter to a jar or airtight container and store it in the refrigerator for freshness.
- The nut butter can be spread on toast, used in recipes, or enjoyed as a dip.

Herbal Tea or Clear Liquid Recipe:

Ingredients:

- Water
- Herbal tea bags (such as chamomile, peppermint, or ginger)
- Clear broths (chicken, beef, vegetable) - store-bought or homemade
- Instructions
- Boil water in a kettle or saucepan.
- Place herbal tea bags (1 bag per cup of water) in a teapot or cup.
- Pour the boiling water over the tea bags.
- Let the tea steep for the recommended time (usually 5-10 minutes), or according to the instructions on the tea packaging.
- Remove the tea bags and discard them.
- If desired, add a sweetener such as honey or sugar to taste.
- Stir well to dissolve the sweetener.
- Allow the tea to cool slightly before serving.
- Serve the herbal tea warm or chilled, depending on your preference.

Avocado Smoothie:

Ingredients:

- 1 ripe avocado
- 1 cup of milk (cow's milk, soy milk, almond milk, etc.)
- 1 tablespoon of honey or maple syrup (optional, for added sweetness)
- Ice cubes (optional, for a chilled and thicker consistency)

Instructions:

- Cut the avocado in half, remove the pit, and scoop out the flesh.
- In a blender, combine the avocado flesh, milk, and sweetener (if using).
- Blend the ingredients on high speed until smooth and creamy.
- If desired, add a few ice cubes to the blender and blend again to achieve a chilled and thicker consistency.
- Taste the smoothie and adjust the sweetness by adding more sweetener if desired.
- Blend briefly to incorporate the added sweetener.
- Pour the avocado smoothie into a glass and serve immediately.

Green Vegetable Juice:

Ingredients:

- 2 cups of mixed green vegetables (such as spinach, kale, cucumber, celery)
- 1 cup of water or vegetable broth
- 1 tablespoon of lemon juice (optional, for added flavor)
- Pinch of salt and pepper

Instructions:

- Wash and prepare the green vegetables by removing any tough stems or leaves.
- Place the green vegetables and water or vegetable broth in a blender.
- Blend on high speed until the mixture becomes smooth and well combined.
- If desired, add lemon juice for a tangy flavor.
- Season with a pinch of salt and pepper to enhance the taste.
- Strain the juice through a fine mesh sieve or cheesecloth to remove any fiber or solids, if desired.
- Pour the green vegetable juice into a glass and serve chilled.

Coconut Milk Pudding:

Ingredients:

- 2 cups of coconut milk
- 1/4 cup of sugar or sweetener of your choice
- 1/4 cup of cornstarch
- 1 teaspoon of vanilla extract (optional, for flavor)

Instructions:

- In a saucepan, combine the coconut milk, sugar, cornstarch, and vanilla extract (if using).
- Place the saucepan over medium heat and whisk continuously until the mixture thickens and comes to a boil.
- Reduce the heat to low and let the pudding simmer for an additional 2 minutes, stirring constantly.
- Remove the saucepan from heat and let the pudding cool slightly.
- Pour the pudding into individual serving cups or a large bowl.
- Cover the pudding with plastic wrap, making sure the wrap touches the surface of the pudding to prevent a skin from forming.
- Chill the pudding in the refrigerator for at least 2 hours or until it is fully set.
- Serve the coconut milk pudding chilled, either on its own or with toppings such as fresh fruits or shredded coconut.

CONCLUSION

The full liquid diet serves as a valuable tool in various medical conditions, post-surgical recovery, and dietary management. It provides individuals with the necessary nutrients while maintaining a liquid consistency, allowing for easy digestion and absorption. Throughout this book, we have explored the definition, purpose, benefits, potential risks, and guidelines for a nutritionally complete full liquid diet.

By understanding the role of a full liquid diet in medical treatment, recovery, and overall health, individuals and healthcare professionals can make informed decisions regarding its implementation. We have examined its differentiation from other dietary plans, identified specific conditions where it is recommended, and delved into the insights provided by medical professionals.

Moreover, we have explored a wide range of full liquid options, including recipes for milk, yogurt, cream-based soups, broths, fruit juices, vegetable juices, protein shakes, gelatin, pudding, fruit smoothies, ice cream or sorbet, fruit purees, vegetable purees, nut butters, and herbal teas or clear liquids. These recipes provide not only nourishment but also variety and enjoyment during the full liquid diet journey.

It is important to note that the full liquid diet should always be followed under the guidance of a healthcare professional and tailored to individual needs and dietary restrictions. It is not meant to be a long-term solution but rather a temporary measure to address specific health concerns.

By adopting a holistic approach to nutrition, incorporating a variety of liquids that meet nutritional requirements, and understanding the principles of a full liquid diet, individuals can successfully navigate this dietary plan and optimize their health and well-being.

Ultimately, the full liquid diet empowers individuals to take charge of their health, providing them with a path towards nourishment, recovery, and a renewed sense of vitality. With the knowledge and resources provided in this book, individuals can embark on their full liquid diet journey with confidence, knowing that they have the tools to make informed choices and achieve their health goals.